CHARIS JAKES

The whole idea about dating

This book was professionally typeset on Reedsy
Find out more at reedsy.com

Contents

1. Dating. 1

2. Self exploration..9

3. Ready for a relationship? 16

4. Basics of dating. 29

1.

2.

3.

One

Dating.

What exactly is dating about?

Dating is the stage of a romantic relationship where two people do things together, usually to see if one of them is a good match for the other in a long-term relationship. It is a form of courtship that involves the couple going to social events by themselves or with others. The terms used to describe dating and the protocols and practices that accompany them vary greatly across cultures, societies, and time periods. Even though the term "dating" is often used loosely to refer to the act of going on dates with other people, it can also refer to a wide range of activities that don't involve going on dates.

During the 20th century, the term "dating" also took on a more casual meaning, referring to a romantic, sexual relationship that goes beyond the initial, trial phase. Despite being informal, this meaning is widely used in formal writing and speech.

Premarital sex has become increasingly common over the past century, beginning with the sexual revolution, despite being taboo for the majority of the world's history. Throughout a greater number of depictions in film, television, and music, sex in a relationship has come to be accepted as a natural progression.

The term "dating" can mean a variety of things, but the most common one is that it refers to a trial period during which two people decide whether or not to move on to a more committed relationship; In this sense, the term "dating" refers to the time when two people are actually together in public, as opposed to the earlier time when they are arranging a date, perhaps through email, text, or phone communication. The term "dating" can also be used to refer to a time in a person's life when they are actively seeking romantic relationships with a variety of people. When two unmarried celebrities are seen together in public, it is common to refer to them as "dating." This means that they were seen together in public, and it is not clear if they are just friends, looking into a more intimate relationship, or romantically involved. When two people have only been out in public a few times but have not yet committed to a relationship, this is a related meaning of the term. Dating, in this sense, is like "being in a committed relationship" in that it is a trial period.

Evaluation

Evaluating one another's suitability as a long-term partner or spouse is one of the primary goals of dating. People who are involved are frequently judged based on their personality, financial situation, and other characteristics, which can hurt feelings and shake confidence. Dating can be very stressful for everyone involved because of the uncertainty of the situation as a whole, the desire to be liked by the other person, and the possibility of being rejected. Dating can be extremely challenging for people with social anxiety disorder, according to some studies.

There is a lot of room for experimentation, and there are numerous sources of advice available, despite the fact that some of what happens on a date is guided by an understanding of fundamental, unspoken rules. Articles in magazines, self-help books, dating coaches, and friends are all sources of advice. Advice can be given about all aspects of dating, including where to go, what to say, what not to say, what to wear, how to end a date, how to flirt, and different. Advice can also be given about how to meet potential partners before a date and how to end a relationship after a date.

Advantages of dating.

1. It brings you joy.

Your happy hormones are released when you are in love with someone. It's not surprising that some people refer to their partners as "happy pills."It shouldn't come as a surprise that your "sweetheart" is the first person you want to help you when you're down or when something is wrong.

2. You feel more confident and secure when you have a partner who supports you.

Not only is it inspiring to have a boyfriend or girlfriend who is supportive, It motivates you to work hard at achieving your goals or passions. You become more confident in your abilities when you have a partner who believes in you, and the desire to impress them motivates you to work harder as well.

3. Your stress levels are lower.

A healthy relationship can help relieve stress. In addition to buffering you from your dramas, your partner can cheer you up when you're feeling down after a difficult workday. You can get more energy by going for a walk or jog in the park at night, going to the movies with a friend, or just talking over a cup of coffee.

4. Someone is honest enough to correct you.

The one who truly cares about you will never allow you to make mistakes. If your partner corrects you whenever you make a mistake, you are heading in the right direction. You can be influenced to be a decent person and citizen by them.

5. You learn more about who you are and who you want to spend the rest of your life with.

Yes, going out on your own will help you learn more about yourself, your personality, and your abilities. However, whenever you are with another person, being in a relationship can also help you learn more about yourself—your social skills, attitude, and true character. In addition, this is the time when you can determine whether or not you really want to spend the rest of your life with the person you are in love with.

6. It teaches you patience and understanding.

Your patience will be severely tested if you spend time with someone who has a different upbringing and personality than you do. Misunderstandings in a relationship are normal, but if you and your partner are willing to work things out, you will soon learn to control your temper and expand your patience and mutual understanding.

7.You learn to be modest.

Humility is one of the keys to a happy, long-lasting relationship. Even if they believe they are not to blame for the conflict, mature couples are forgiving, willing to make mistakes, and capable of apologizing to one another.

8.It broadens your perspective.

You must respect your partner's thoughts and accept that you may not always be right in a relationship. It opens your eyes to the fact that different people typically have different perspectives on the world, and it's possible that your partner has different perspectives than you do. If you want a happy relationship, you should know better than to demand your partner's opinions.

9.Someone will look after you and check on you.

Having someone, other than your mother, who looks out for your welfare is one of the practical advantages of being in a relationship. Someone will check to see if you have eaten or are safe at home late at night. In addition, when you were ill, someone would cook you your favorite meals and ensure that you had taken your medications.

10.Being healthy is encouraged more.

Certainly, one of your goals as you work together to plan for the future is to stay healthy to avoid costly hospitalizations and other terrible consequences of having a sick family member. You'll notice that you want to exercise more often and that your food choices are healthier. It will also be easier to give up bad habits like smoking and drinking alcohol.

11.Future planning becomes a team effort.

When you are single, you are free to fantasize about your goals and future family. However, you are able to practically begin planning for those objectives only when you are in a committed relationship. By moving in that direction now, you become partners in accountability for ensuring that those plans will be carried out.

12.Your circle of friends and family expand.

As you enter the world of your partner, being committed to a relationship allows you to broaden your social circle. You get to know his or her friends as well as his or her family and begin to develop a relationship with them.

13.You will be assisted in becoming a better person by someone.

If it helps you become a more mature person, you can say that you are in a healthy relationship overall. You and your partner need to work together to improve one another's physical, emotional, financial, mental, and spiritual stability. This occurs as you both humbly acknowledge your shortcomings and work to improve them.

14.You discover what it truly means to be in love.

A healthy and long-lasting relationship is the result of genuine love. By prioritizing your partner's needs, it will teach you to be selfless. In addition, as you give without expecting anything in return, you discover the meaning of unconditional love.

Two

Self exploration.

Life moves quickly. There are tasks to complete, errands to run, and commitments to keep. It's possible that self-discovery is the last thing on our minds.

We rarely have time to think about the kind of life we really want because of our busy schedules. While waiting in line at the grocery store, do you think about who you are? Probably not. Finding the space to discover and become our most authentic selves can be challenging. However, there are numerous advantages that make the effort worthwhile.

If you're wondering how to start self-discovery, know that making a commitment is the first step. You will need to be focused, take action, and prioritize your needs throughout your journey. Keep in mind that you can't change anything without working hard.

Are you prepared to learn how to begin your journey of self-discovery?To begin, let's define what self-discovery is.

What exactly is self-discovery?

Understanding one's true self is the process of self-discovery. Your beliefs, requirements, and even the foods you like and don't like. Some of these things about yourself may have come to you naturally over time. However, we have a tendency, for a lot of people, to lose touch with our values and to conceal our own motives and preferences, even from ourselves. Your life can be changed by delving deeper into self-discovery.

Knowing your personality type or your favorite dish is one thing. But the first step toward true self-discovery is to look at your life and decide what makes you happy and what doesn't. What will make your life more joyful? What motivates you to get out of bed each day?

Finding your life's purpose and being your authentic self at work and in your personal life will be easier once you know more about yourself. You will gain insight into who you are by comprehending what has been lacking in your life.

However, don't think you can complete this journey in a day. Self-discovery is a process that never ends. It requires you to examine every aspect of your life and take the time to think about it. To stick with the process, you'll need courage and resilience because looking within may reveal things about yourself that are hard to accept.

Self-knowledge, also known as self-awareness, is essential for discovering one's inner self. The term "self-knowledge" typically refers to an understanding of one's own thoughts, feelings, and aspirations. Emotional regulation will improve if you have more of this in your life. Both your personal and professional relationships will benefit from this, as will your ability to manage stress.

Empathy, self-control, creativity, and self-esteem all benefit from gaining a better understanding of how your mind works. As a result, your honesty will grow even more.

Learning how to begin a journey of self-discovery has numerous advantages. The most important thing is to start by taking the first step.

New call to action: How to start a journey of self-discovery You might be afraid to start a journey of self-discovery. How exactly do you begin? There are no predetermined steps to self-discovery. This means that you can begin with any action that feels right to you. Keep the momentum going because it is admirable to have the courage to start this journey.

To help you figure out who you are, here are 10 suggestions:

* Make sure you surround yourself with people who support you.

* Learn from your mistakes and move on.

* Think back to your childhood and connect with your inner child again. *Be curious and ask questions.

* Create habits that support your personal growth and goals.

* Practice positive self-talk and reward yourself for your wins. *Discovering your true self will help you feel more confident in your ability to make decisions.

* Take risks and try new things. *Focus on your passions and what excites you.

    * Understand your strengths and consider how you can apply them everywhere.

Because self-discovery helps you gain a profound understanding of yourself, this holds true for all aspects of your life.You'll know what's best for you than anyone else.

Here are five things to keep in mind as you work to become more self-aware:

* Focus on what gives you energy and what drains it.
    * Visualize the person you want to be.
    * Follow where your passions and interests lead you.
    * Let go of your inner critic and any self-doubt.
    * Choose a life of meaning and be purposeful with your actions.

Importance of self-discovery.

We benefit from self-discovery because it enables us to have more meaningful lives. When you understand yourself, you can better take care of yourself. In addition, if you are in touch with your authentic self, you might be able to find a career that gives you more satisfaction.

Additionally, you are more likely to succeed if you choose a career path that truly piques your interest.

You might discover that, despite being an introvert, you are also a people person. It's always important to take care of our social health, but maybe you need more social connections than you thought.

Additionally, this gives you a better understanding of your desired future. You can plan a future that meets your needs and supports your well-being by understanding yourself. You won't be able to live your life to the fullest and with the most passion.

Let's say you reflect and discover that the projects you lead at work are your favorites. This probably indicates that you are gifted in leadership or that you enjoy it. In light of this, you can work toward becoming a manager. You'll have a better understanding of your career path and a job that you enjoy doing more.

Additionally, strengths and weaknesses can be identified when one is aware of themselves. Perhaps you are an expert in compassion, empathy, or mindfulness.

Alternately, you might be an exceptional author or speaker. The best way to find out is to get started on your journey of self-discovery.

Additionally, this procedure can assist you in identifying areas of improvement. Taking the time to reflect on yourself will demonstrate that you need to improve your communication skills, for example.

Your journey of self-discovery will have an impact on the lives of others as well. In your social life, you can use your newly sharpened skills to build stronger relationships. You will become a better friend, coworker, and family member as a result of this authenticity.

Five advantages of self-discovery.

The path to self-discovery can take various forms for numerous individuals. However, it has advantages that assist you in becoming your authentic self for everyone.

To put that into perspective, consider the following five advantages that can result from discovering who you are:

1. When you have a better understanding of your core values and what you want out of life, your relationships will thrive and be healthier. You will be able to resolve deeper issues and identify toxic traits, whether they are yours or not. If you are then more open and honest, you can improve your social health.

2. You'll have less self-doubt because you'll know that mistakes sometimes happen because we're human rather than criticizing every mistake you make. You are not a bad person

because of it. Additionally, as you gain self-awareness, you will learn to avoid certain errors. The first step in avoiding repeat mistakes is to comprehend why you made them.

3. You'll be more creative because you'll be able to share your feelings with others and become more creative. But if you don't know who you are, how can you express yourself? You can discover your identity and learn how to express it through self-reflection.

4. You'll be better able to concentrate on what you really want because the ongoing process of figuring out who you are requires you to be dedicated and focused. With a stronger sense of self in mind, this practice will assist you in setting and achieving objectives. You can plan a future that reflects your true self.

5. You will feel more confident in yourself. Believing in yourself and your abilities can have an effect on both your personal and professional lives. You will approach new experiences as a whole person with increased self-assurance, not as someone who shies away from challenges or change. In addition, your self-confidence will continue to rise as you begin your journey toward self-improvement.

Three

Ready for a relationship?

Are you ready for a relationship?

The concept of being "ready" for a relationship is widespread and ambiguous. An all-purpose justification for any number of reasons why a person might or might not want a romantic partner, "Readiness" is a well-worn T-shirt that people put on and take off repeatedly throughout their dating lives. When someone says, "I'm just not ready for a relationship right now," it's often unclear what they mean. And the conclusion—there won't be a relationship—is just as significant as the deeper meaning of that statement. It is a cliche that is simple to cover up, to use as a cover for the true reasons behind a breakup, and to prevent self-examination from bringing up more difficult emotions.

Some people view "readiness" as an external metric: are my current circumstances favorable to dating?Others view it as internal: Am I willing to be observed? Can I deal with the difficulties of a relationship?

Externally, being prepared is frequently discussed in terms of timing; "it's not a great time for me right now" is a common way to convey unpreparedness without explicitly stating it. A person may be too busy, uncertain about the future, or recently separated to commit to a new partner. We are told that just finding the right person is not enough. Also, it needs to be the right time.

To a certain extent, this may be true. Time can be a problem. It doesn't have to stop someone from getting together; It's just something to think about.

How to determine whether someone likes you.

I'm sure you've asked yourself and probably someone close to you, "Do they really like me?" when you first meet someone, and "how can I be sure?"

Hints that someone is interested in you;

They are consistent and always have time to see you.

In fact, they don't just find the time; they make it happen! This usually means that they are interested in you and want to spend as much time as possible with you. The fact that they consistently show up on time, among other things is also a positive sign because it demonstrates their effort and genuine desire to be there.

When you first start dating or discover that another person in your friend group or at work likes you, this becomes very clear. Is there anyone who will always want to be in your current location? tries to get to know you? has time to speak with you?

Be on the lookout for those who show up strong at first because they may have an avoidant attachment—they want to be with someone but back off when they get close to them because they feel uncomfortable. This This could be a red flag, and you may need to hold back a little bit if they initially appear overly enthusiastic hen you get around to talking about their previous relationships, you should be able to determine whether this is the case.

** Being in energy.*

When When someone likes you, they tend to lean toward you subconsciously when you're together. It creates a physical closeness that demonstrates that they are attracted to you and drawn into your energy.

If you find yourself moving away, it could mean that you don't find them as attractive and that their energy is making you feel like your space is being invaded. You shouldn't ignore this warning. It could be because you're aware of something you need to back away from subconsciously, or it could be your own avoidance mechanisms work

They want to talk.

If someone wants to learn more about you, they'll start a conversation to find out what you like to do, what interests you, where you've been, and anything else they can think of to keep the conversation. When someone likes you, this is one of the most common behaviors they exhibit. They want to see how well you get along with each other by finding things you share.

If someone is shy or struggles with self-worth and confidence, this may not occur; therefore, even if you like them, don't dismiss them. They will open up and engage more after a few meetings. They probably aren't interested if they don't.

If they keep talking about you, your past, and the difficult times in your life, or if they talk a lot about their own problems, this is a sign to leave.

There is a deeper interest in

Curiosity is a fascinating quality—provided, of course, that you are not a Out! You want to learn more about something in order to have a better understanding of the situation when you become curious about it. This is made worse in a romantic situation because your brain is trying to learn more about why it was triggered and becomes extremely interested in the person who caused it.

To satisfy that curiosity, it will continue to ask questions. Your friends are likely to inquire about them as well once they meet the person who is interested in you.

Take note of the caveat to this in the preceding section: be wary of where their curiosity might be.

** They will smile a lot.*

When they are drawn to you, they will look at you and smile. They are definitely in a good spot around you if you notice that they are still smiling and glancing away.

The rate at which you smile increases and also grows larger, broader, and longer when you are around someone you are drawn to. The light in their eyes, the raised cheekbones, and the wrinkles around the eyes are all indications that the smile is genuine.

** Pay attention to how they feel when you're around them.*

Being around someone you like can affect how they feel physically.

They feel anxious as a result, which is good stress in this instance. The release of adrenaline and other hormones will accelerate your heart rate and circulate blood throughout your body, possibly resulting in blushing or even more sweating. It is something that people can't help but do, and it will affect how much energy they give you.

It should feel like they're excited to be around you, but it could also mean they want to get away from you. Keep an eye out for the difference when taking into consideration the other things I've mentioned.

** They remember the "small stuff.*

If someone remembers something you said, even if only briefly, and then comes back to it later, they are probably interested. They clearly listened to what you said, so it's important for them to remember it.

Your brain will allow you to recall things that are important to you because of "selective filtering."If your brain is telling you that something is important, it usually means that you care about it, so the other person probably cares about you as well

Time for a caveat: there are people who keep things about you because they think it's important to remember later and use against you. You can rest assured that they are interested if it is the small things you have shared rather than personal information because this clearly does not relate to.

In conclusion, if you want to know if someone is interested in you but doesn't explicitly state it, look for clues? Although they may not display all of them, a few of them convey that they wish to get to know Keep. Keep in mind that it can be difficult for some people to come out, so if you like them, show them the signs instead.Or, simply inform them.

If you struggle with acceptance or fear of rejection and want to create a little more certainty about someone before letting your feelings show, I know it can be difficult to do this, but recognizing the signs will help you determine whether or not it is safe to reciprocate.

Be aware of the warning signs as Some.Some people have issues that make them want you to be interested in them just to get what they need, or they know what they want but won't let themselves have it.

Take the pressure off of yourself by going out, having fun, relaxing, being yourself, and seeing where the world of relationships takes you. Always keep your mind on the person you want in your Treat yourself well.

How to contact someone.

The truth: It's extremely nerve-wracking to ask someone out. Putting yourself out there, no matter how confident you are, is risky because it hurts to be turned down. In point of fact, a slew of recent studies have demonstrated that some of the neural and —neurochemical substrates that are shared by physical pain and social pain—the emotional response to being rejected or ostracized by others—are actually the same. To put it another way, when you stub your toe and the person you like turns you down, similar processes are taking place in your brain.

This is largely why it hurts to be rejected; it hurts so much that you might avoid asking people out or act so casual and hesitant that the person you're asking out doesn't know if it's a date or not.

This is not the way to act when you ask someone out, you need to be direct, bold, and confident Additionally, you must fully comprehend and believe that rejection is not fatal. It's actually beneficial to be rejected. You'd learn to respect other people's boundaries and avoid wasting time with people who don't want to be with you.

Don't worry if asking someone out sounds confusing or terrifying. You can find everything you need right

Everything you need to know about how to ask someone out without worrying about their response.

I have the advice you need to get that date—or at least try to—over text, phone, or in person.

How to ask someone out without being strange is as follows.

1.Don't overthink

When it comes to making the first move, we can be our own worst fear. Fear of being rejected is one of the most common issues men have in relationships.

No one wants to look foolish or be rejected for being ourselves. In addition, it's hard to feel good when rejected. We avoid taking healthy risks like putting ourselves out there because of our anxiety. This way of thinking happens to keep our egos safe and from harm.

You will psych yourself out if you get too caught up in thinking about you. You read into things when you build everything up in your head, text for days on end, and don't make concrete plans. We do it all.

Don't give it too much thought or make it harder than it needs to be "Ask if [they] want to have dinner or drinks."

Simply go for it! Awesome if they say Yes. You didn't waste more time than you had to if they do.

2. Keeping things simple and straightforward.

When it comes to asking someone keep things simple and straightforward. If you do this, you will irritate the other person and run the risk of falling into a deep misunderstanding.

"When you ask a question like "Want to hang?," don't be vague. When asking them out, be specific. For instance, "Do you have time for dinner on Tuesday?" It demonstrates that you care about them as a person rather than just as someone to "hang out with. Dates are Dates. Be unapologetic and bold about it. Amateurs should avoid caginess.

3. Don't make elaborate plans for your dates.

There seems to be a lot of pressure to "stand out" or to be interesting. To be memorable, you don't have to take them to the zoo, ice skating, skydiving, or deep sea fishing if you have the personality. Be authentic.

We know this sounds corny, but many guys try to be someone they aren't, especially those who are afraid of being rejected. They act as though they're some sophisticated, clever womanizer they think women

Warning: This is a spoiler: (Most do not.) Be different from those guys. According to Shamyra Howard, LCSW, a sex and relationship expert, "authenticity is the best game you can bring." Don't portray yourself as you think you should; It's best to be who you really are. This is not the time to try to fool around. You want to be appreciated for who you are. In addition, how much longer will you be able to maintain facade of being someone else?

4. Pay close attention to the response when you ask via text.

They they aren't necessarily uninterested in it if you don't get a definitive " Yes." Pay close attention to how they respond if this is the case. They are not interested if they are busy and do not offer you another option. They are interested, but they can't make the day you suggested if they offer an alternate time or day to meet. Don't take it as a rejection if they try to reschedule. Give them an opportunity to bring it about. Well, you have your answer if they don't. "If they don't respond, you can try again on a different day." Let them go and move on if they don't respond the second time.

In fact, it's pretty easy: You'll get along with anyone who wants to go out with you. They won't if they don't. Put in the work, wait for the same in return, and if you don't get it, move on with your life.

5. Start by making small talk if you're actually ask

Meeting someone in person and asking them out (we know, what) has its own regulations. Do not simply approach a cute person and ask them out. Make small talk to find out what interests each other. Watch how they respond."For instance, you should move on if you approach someone and they do not respond, are short with you, or move further away. If not, depending on where you approach them, talk about something that they might be interested in.

Based on your environment, interpret the situation. If you're waiting for a coffee, ask them about their favorite beverage or whether they've tried the new seasonal drink. Keep going if they engage with you. Inquire about their name, occupation, Simply avoid being creepy about it.

It takes self-awareness to pay attention to body language and the vibe you're getting. She is actually preventing you from seeing her by crossing her arms and legs. Give her a break. Don't ask her out if she doesn't fully turn to face you because this probably means she doesn't want to talk to you. Now, she is interested if she has shifted her position to face you directly, is smiling, and making eye contact. Request a coffee date with her this week if you still have the go-ahead.

If you do get rejected, consider the following: What then? Seriously, how will this affect you for the rest of your life?

It is not you. "You might have ended up with someone who wasn't a good match for you if rejection didn't exist.

6. Accept it if you ask her out and she says no.

Don't try to persuade her to change their mind for the love of God. Some classic romantic films, like The Notebook, teach men that persistence is a sign of love and devotion, but it's not. It scares me. It actually violates consent and is a major deterrent.

Four

Basics of dating.

How to Start a Relationship:

1. Know What You Want (and Are Willing to Give).

Relationships and dating are social exchanges. They are an industry. Past the sensations of adoration - individuals are hoping to get some kind of needs met. Their partners are also.

Despite this, many people date without knowing anyone. They don't plan anything. As a result, they frequently do not receive what they require and have to content themselves with what they are offered by others or nothing at all. After all, if a person doesn't know what they want, they shouldn't be surprised if they don't get it in a mysterious way.

As a result, it helps to know what you want before dating. Knowing what you will do for others in return is also essential. As you interact, be aware of what you are trading. Success in dating is primarily based on being clear about those issues.

2. Look and act your best.

Everyone wants to be loved for who they really are. They want other people to see them as they really are. Actually, dating doesn't work that way. No, you don't have to be a supermodel or a bodybuilder to meet someone. However, it is unrealistic to expect others to search for the "real them" inside if they are horribly grumpy or smell like an old gym bag. Although there may be more to a book than just its cover, the cover is what initially entices readers to read it (or put it on the shelf).

Therefore, it pays to put your best foot forward when dating. Again, the plastic surgeon is unnecessary. However, taking care of one's appearance, dressing well, smelling good, and remaining healthy all contribute significantly. Similarly, a pleasant disposition and a hint of masculinity or femininity (depending on who you want to attract) are very powerful. To be honest, people enjoy being around people who are pleasant in appearance and disposition. Paying attention to these little things can make a big difference.

3. Learn to read body language and use it.

Most relationships fail because people don't read the signs. There are a million nonverbal cues that people use every day."Please talk to me," "you're cute," and "pay attention here" are common phrases. It is evident that others yell "get lost," "not you," or "today is a bad day."

Unfortunately, the majority of people are so clueless about body language that they miss invitations (or warning signs) from others. They also fail to convey the appropriate signals on their own. Don't be surprised if the cute person you're crushing on doesn't come up to you and say hello if you're walking around tense and grumpy like you want to wring someone's neck!

Therefore, learning to read and respond appropriately is the key. Additionally, it is crucial to pay attention to what other people are saying through their actions rather than their words. Knowing who to flirt with and ask out will be much easier if you master these skills. It will also assist in attracting other people.

4. Be Brave:

"Fortune favors the brave," Dating also rewards bravery. Sadly, many people avoid danger, are afraid, and are unsure. Because of this, many other people miss out on getting to know that special someone because they were too shy to say hello.

In all honesty, dating is a numbers game. Before you find a real princess or prince, you will probably have to kiss a lot of frogs. Most likely, your first love will not be your last. As a result, getting the love you want is more likely to come your way if you are more at ease socializing, making new friends, and dealing with rejection.

In general, courage is directly related to dating success. The key is to learn to date without fear, approach others with confidence, and accept rejection. Even if you're looking for the "one and only," you'll probably have to sort through a lot of them to find them. Therefore, engaging in social activities can be beneficial.

5. You have a better chance of getting what you want if you ask for it, whether it's on your first or 100th date.

However, a lot of people just sit around and hope. They hope that they will be noticed. They anticipate being asked out by someone. However, hope is not very effective, persuasive, or even influential.

In a strange twist, asking is very successful. One study, for instance, found that when a stranger of average attractiveness asked them out on a date, 68% of single men and 43% of single women said yes. This finding has been confirmed by others.

Women, who frequently adopt a more passive dating style, may benefit most from this strategy. Again, studies show that if they just ask for what they want, they usually get what they want. Therefore, do not remain aloof. You never know what you'll get if you ask.

Conclusion.

Dating doesn't have to be a mystery. It does not even have to be difficult. It only requires a little bit of thought, effort, and bravery!

So, just follow the steps above if you're having trouble dating or making it too complicated. Simpler is better. Go socialize. Expect a fair trade with your offer. Make your demands known. You will be pleasantly surprised if you put some effort into those areas...

Healthy Relationships.

What Does It Mean to Have a Happy Relationship?

Honesty, trust, respect, and open communication are essential components of healthy relationships, which necessitate effort and compromise on the part of both partners. There is no power imbalance. Partners honor each other's independence, share decisions, and can make their own choices without fear of retaliation. There is no stalking or refusing to let go of the other partner when a relationship ends.

Healthy relationships are characterized by;

* Respect for one another's space and privacy. You don't have to spend every day with your partner.

* Your partner encourages you to engage in enjoyable activities and spend time alone with friends.

* You feel comfortable talking about your thoughts and worries with your partner.

* Your partner doesn't force you to have sex or do things that make you feel uncomfortable, so you feel physically safe.

* When there are disagreements or conflicts, your partner respects your wishes and feelings, and you can negotiate and come to an agreement.

A healthy relationship is built on the following elements:

1. Boundaries: You and your partner are able to meet each other's needs in a way that works for both of you.

2. Communication: Even if you don't agree, you and your partner can talk about your feelings in a way that makes the other person feel safe, heard, and not judged.

3. Trust:Since couples can rely on one another, they are able to be vulnerable with one another and build trust over time.

4. Consent:Giving consent means that you are okay with what is happening and that no one is forcing you to do anything you don't want to do. This expression is most frequently used when engaging in sexual activity. At any time, consent can be given and taken back, and giving consent once does not guarantee that you will give consent again.

By looking at the other sections to your left, you can see how these things go together.

Please keep in mind that attempting to enforce boundaries, open communication, trust, and other healthy behaviors in some abusive relationships could put your safety at risk. Keep in mind that power and control are at the heart of abuse, and an abusive person may be unwilling to relinquish their hold over you.

BOUNDARIES.

A boundary is similar to a line. There are things on one side that you are okay with, and there are things on the other side that you are not okay with, aren't ready for, or make you feel uncomfortable. You need to know where your line needs to be drawn because everyone sees this line differently. A way to teach your partner about your needs and let you know when something doesn't feel right is to set boundaries. You are permitted to prioritize your needs over those of another person, particularly if those needs make you uncomfortable.

Step 1: What boundaries do you have?

Consider each of these subcategories and consider what they mean for your relationship.

* Physical: Are you okay with showing affection in public? Is it uncomfortable for you to be affectionate? Do you despise or adore being tickled by your partner? Do you require a lot of time alone? Learn more about abuse and physical boundaries.

*Emotional: Do you have the ability to express your feelings right away or do you require some time to consider them? Do you need your partner to be there for you whenever you need them? When are you ready to express your love for me? Learn more about abuse and emotional boundaries.

*Sexual: Are you okay with getting physical right away or do you need to get to know your partner for a while before doing anything sexual? What kind of sexual activity can you tolerate? Learn more about abuse and sexual boundaries.

*Digital: Do you post information about your relationship? Is it acceptable for your spouse to use your phone? Would you like to exchange passwords? Learn more about abuse and digital boundaries.

*Material: Do you enjoy sharing your possessions?Do you mind paying for your partner or the other way around?

*Spiritual: Do you prefer to practice your religion alone or with a partner?Is it necessary for your partner to share your beliefs, or can they be different as long as they respect yours? Are you planning to have sex before getting married?

Step 2: communicating your boundaries to your partner.

You are not required to sit down with your partner and make a list of everything that makes you feel uneasy; however, you are required to be open and honest. If you are a virgin and don't want to have sex until you are ready, for example, some of these things might come up early in the relationship. If your partner wants to share passwords after six months of dating, for instance, some of these issues may not arise for some time. Talk about your needs when they differ from your partner's; You don't have to explain anything. A healthy relationship necessitates having difficult conversations, despite the awkwardness. Trust is built when your partner respects you and listens to you.

Step 3: knowing when a boundary has been crossed.

Even after you've spoken with your partner, boundaries can still be violated from time to time; This is where self-trust comes into play. You might be depressed, anxious, or irate, or you might not even know what you're feeling. Always follow your heart. It probably isn't if something doesn't feel right to you.

Step 4: Responding.

Have an open discussion with your partner if they have crossed a line that you didn't know existed. It might be as straightforward as saying, "Hey, I really don't like it when you _________."I'm really uneasy about this. Do you think you could _______ next time? Although reaching an agreement that meets both of your needs may require some back and forth, your relationship will be strengthened as a result.

Abuse may occur if a boundary has been crossed despite your prior declaration of those boundaries. When your partner uses physical force to coerce you into doing something you don't want to do, for example, you may be crossing a line that should be obvious. However, it can also be less obvious, such as when your partner coerces you into doing something, begs you until you comply, or threatens to break up with you unless you comply.

COMMUNICATION

Because it enables you to share who you are and what you require from the people around you, open and honest communication is an essential component of every relationship. Misunderstandings are all too common, and they frequently result in conflicts, misunderstandings, and hurt feelings. You can talk to your partner honestly with the help of these tips.

> **Speaking:** Be honest and open about your feelings; Inform them if you don't understand something; make use of "I statements" to avoid giving the impression that you are attacking or blaming the other person ("I feel that..."); Be sincere, even if you think the other person won't like to hear how you really feel; When you've done something wrong or hurt someone, say sorry; Include something positive when discussing something negative.

>**Listening:** Put your phone away and pay attention to what the other person is saying; instead of only considering how to respond, pay attention to what they are saying; Before you say anything, wait for them to finish speaking; Use phrases like "interesting" to indicate that you understand what they are saying; If you don't understand something, ask questions to avoid misunderstanding; Don't leave them hanging (advise them that you need to think about what they said before responding); Be ready to hear something you don't like, and give it some serious thought before responding.

How you act: Contact one another; toward them; Lean in and give them your full attention as they speak.

Electronic Communication: Don't discuss important matters via text or online. Focus on the conversation at hand rather than getting sidetracked by other things or having multiple conversations when online; Let the other person know if you are unable to respond so you don't leave them hanging.

When and where to have a crucial discussion: If you were in a fight, talk about something important when you are calm, or take some time to calm down. Discuss your concerns before they develop into issues and become more serious. To be honest about your feelings, ensure that you are speaking in private.

Be careful when using these suggestions and check out our "Get Help" section if you think your partner might be emotionally abusing you or doesn't do these things.

TRUST.

Building trust can take time. Even though it can be difficult to trust someone, especially if you haven't trusted them before, you can't hold your current partner responsible for something they did.

Several strategies for fostering trust include:

1. <u>Be dependable</u>: Would they be there for you if you needed a ride home from school or someone to listen to you when you were having a bad day?Would you support them?

2. <u>Maintain boundaries:</u> Do you get respect from your partner when you tell them something makes you feel uncomfortable? Does it apply to both sides?

3. <u>Be sincere</u>: Does your partner share their feelings with you instead of keeping their feelings to themselves? Do you try to talk things out with your partner and share your feelings?Would you tell your partner if you made a mistake? Would your spouse inform you?

Don't just talk the talk; actually do the work: Say what you mean, do what you say.

CONSENT.

Consent is a verbal or nonverbal declaration by two people that they are both enthusiastically and clearly willing to engage in sexual activity. Consent does not include silence or resistance. Some people, such as those who are intoxicated, asleep, or unconscious, and some people with intellectual disabilities, are unable to consent. Active communication and knowing that only one person has the right to revoke consent are essential components of consent. This indicates that consent can be given to one activity—kissing—but not to another—sex. Similar to sex, consent ought to be about respecting one another's right to make their own decisions regarding their bodies.

Consent can be obtained easily:It all comes down to communication. Before having sex, you can talk about boundaries, but you should also check in with a simple, "Is this okay?" every so often to make sure that everyone involved is happy with the situation.

What not to do in a happy relationship.

1. If you don't want the relationship to end, treat your partner as you did at the beginning.

When you first start dating someone, you put in a lot of effort to win them over and impress them.It won't fade or become repetitive if you treat them the same throughout the relationship.

2. Don't give up on your partner.

It's easy to forget what it was like before someone entered your life when they become a part of your routine. You become at ease. Things get used to you. You lose the ability to appreciate what you have when you become too used to having someone.

3. Do learn to make concessions when necessary.

Learn to simply say yes without adding anything else. You won't get into silly fights.

4. Don't let your insecurity or jealousy take over.

Yes, they will be sexy, and their ex-partners might come back and blow up their phone. They are attractive to a wide range of people. However, when jealousy strikes, what you're really saying to your partner is that you don't trust yourself enough to keep you.

5. Learn to choose your battles carefully.

There will be things that require fighting for. Things you really care about and believe in, but the most intelligent people know when to fight and when to just agree with something even when they don't agree with it.

6. Never stop surprising your significant other.

Never stop attempting to keep things interesting and that fire burning. It all comes down to the small acts of kindness you show to others.

7. Do set reasonable goals for them.

Consider the questions you ask? Is what you want the relationship to be based on reality or a fantasy? Reverse the roles and consider whether or not you would be able to cope with their demands and whether or not you could.In addition, are you already carrying out that?

8. Don't let your emotions and feelings build up.

When you allow negative emotions to build up, they will all come out at the wrong time at the wrong time. Take difficult feelings as they arise and deal with them immediately.

9. Give yourself permission to be vulnerable.

Letting someone into every aspect of who you are is the only way to truly connect emotionally. People who recognize that vulnerability is not a sign of weakness have the best relationships.

10. If you're unhappy with something they're doing, don't blame them all.

If they aren't doing what you want them to do, ask yourself if you're doing enough on your end to get them to want to. Are you providing them with the same level of security as they do, if you want them to be more spontaneous? If you want them to put a little more effort into the physical aspects of your relationships, you are building their confidence and giving them the impression that they are the most attractive person so that they can confidently do something different. Parts of your relationships that aren't where you want them to be are never the fault of just one person.

11. When you need to, give each other some space.

Don't bother checking on them because Saturday is for the boys. On a Friday night, let her go out with her girlfriends as late as she wants. It's important to have a life apart, no matter how much time you spend together.

12. Don't put your happiness in their hands.

You cannot attribute your happiness solely to other people.

13. Do aid them in achieving their objectives.

Encourage them. Support them. Encourage them to reach their goals. Having someone who believes you can do anything is the best approach.

14. Do not attempt to change them.

You might be pleased with the things they could enhance. But if you're unhappy with yourself, don't try to make them into someone they aren't. You don't deserve them if you're trying to change them.

15. Do aid in making them feel safe.

It is your responsibility to make them feel safe, and they ought to be as self-assured as you are.

16. Do not conceal anything from them.

Even if it hurts, be open and honest with them. The truth will always come out, and if you try to hide it, it will make the person even more hurt.

17. Don't ignore them.

Build them up as much as possible. It is intended that your relationship together will be your healthiest one.

18. Don't let the fact that you have them convince you to let go.

Keep going to the gym. Nonetheless, eat well. Take care of yourself, though. Keeping them will be more difficult than getting them. Additionally, you must take care of yourself not for them but rather because you are deserving of being at your most self-assured in front of them.

19. Do establish connections with their family.

Having relationships with their family is essential, even those that you dislike. Never force them to choose between you and them, either.

20. Don't blame them for your past.

It is not their fault that someone has abused you in the past. They have nothing to do with your trust issues. Open up to them about it so they can understand, but don't let them down because you have past experiences that have made you feel insecure.

21. Give them a chance.

It's split 50/50. You don't deserve them if you let them do more than you can handle on your own. Additionally, the right person will respect you and meet you right there, so even if you're working your asses off to maintain this relationship, it will fail.

22.We are wary of the ammunition you use when fighting.

You will regret using something they told you in confidence in a fight. Remember that you care about this person, so no matter how enraged you are, your rage will pass, but the things you say when you're enraged cannot be forgotten.

23. Do strengthen them.

If you're in the right relationship, your positive influence will help them grow into a person twice as big as they are now.

24. Remember important dates.

She says that she cares about what you do, not what we do, and she wants you to surprise her on your anniversary. Anniversaries, Birthdays, Even when women claim that it isn't, it still matters to them.

25. Do give the impression that you are a little bit interested in what they care about.

Put on your best smile and do whatever makes them happy, even if you despise what they care about. Remember that you care about them. You never know, you might like this new thing you've never tried.

26. Don't discount their aspirations.

They won't need that from you because everyone else in the world will have enough doubt about them. Even if you are the only one cheering, they need you to stand by their side and be their cheerleader.

27. Help them learn and forgive them.

Nobody is flawless. They will annoy and irritate you, and there will be times when you wonder why you are with this person who makes you crazy. However, when they make a mistake and apologize, Help them gain knowledge and move on.

28. Don't look for something sneakily.

Don't look at their computer or phone. You will discover something you dislike. There are things about even the best relationships that you will question if you find them. And you'll discover it. And you won't be happy about it. Trust is the fundamental foundation of every relationship. You must have faith that they will treat you with respect even when you are not present.

29. Do tell them every day how much you love them.

Never skip a day without uttering those three words.

30. Avoid hurting their feelings.

Don't look for something better when you already have something and someone that are good. Learn to value what you already have. Learn that the most satisfying relationships are those in which you never give up on one another.

UNHEALTHY RELATIONSHIPS.

Relationships that aren't healthy can have a big effect on your health, happiness, and overall well-being. The issue is that while some relationships are unmistakably toxic or even abusive, others can be much more subtle and difficult to spot.

Even though no relationship is perfect, it's important to be able to spot the warning signs of one and know how to fix it or end it.

How to tell if you're in an unhealthy relationship is the subject of this chapter, which also covers some of the most common characteristics. It also talks about what you can do to improve your relationship and when you should get professional help.

Unhealthy relationships share a number of common traits. Each relationship is unique and may evolve over time. Unhealthy relationships typically share a few crucial characteristics.

Tension, conflict, and stress tend to rise in relationships marked by these dynamics and issues. This is true for romantic relationships, but unhealthy patterns can also have an impact on other types of relationships, such as those with family, friends, and coworkers.

Control One person may attempt to exert control over the other person's life in unhealthy relationships. This can be done by intimidating the person, but it can also be done by using other methods of manipulation. Sometimes the person may act in ways that make them appear to be very affectionate and loving. In fact, the purpose of these actions is to keep an eye on the other person and prevent them from doing things or going places they can't control.

Isolating a person from friends and family is another way to control behavior. It might also entail cutting off communication, restricting financial access, or making it difficult to leave the situation.

Possession and jealousy are other forms of control. When someone tries to control what you do, when they lash out at you when they become upset, or when they accuse you of infidelity, both of these feelings are unhealthy, even though they are common human experiences.

Identifying the Warning Signs of This Dating Situation.

A Lack of Trust.

relationship lack of trust is often a sign of unhealthy relationships. You might think you have to keep certain things from your partner, or you might think they keep certain things from you a lot.

Both partners in a relationship must engage in self-disclosure in a manner that is reciprocal for healthy trust to develop. This requires you to reveal information about yourself over time as the relationship leads to emotional intimacy and closeness are facilitated by the process of sharing and listening. However, you are unlikely to share your innermost thoughts, feelings, or memories with another person if you believe you cannot trust them.

Your overall attachment style may have an impact on your level of trust with your partner. These patterns of behavior are often formed in childhood through interactions and experiences with caregivers; however, even after you reach adulthood, these patterns continue to influence how you respond to romantic relationships.

It may be difficult for you to trust your romantic partners if you have a history of not being able to rely on the people you should be able to trust the most.

In unhealthy relationships, disrespect can manifest itself in a number of different ways. It could mean that one person treats the other person with contempt. In other instances, it may entail openly ridiculing or making fun of the other person's opinions or interests.

This disrespect can frequently feel like rejection, which can cause a variety of feelings, including hurt feelings, shame, guilt, loneliness, embarrassment, and social anxiety.

Inadequate communication.

Effective communication is essential to any relationship that is healthy. Patterns of poor communication are often a sign of unhealthy relationships. To avoid confronting issues in the relationship, this might entail not talking about them, avoiding difficult topics, expecting the other person to be able to read your mind, not listening, becoming defensive, or stalling.

Recap: Controlling behaviors, mistrust, disrespect, and poor communication are some of the common traits that are frequently seen in unhealthy relationships.

Communication style has been shown to be a key predictor of divorce and has more of an impact on marital success than commitment, stress, and personality.

Signs That You Are in a Unhealthy Relationship.

Relationships frequently develop, shift, and occasionally break up over time. When things are going well, a relationship may be mostly healthy, but adding stressors can make things harder. As a response, people may resort to unhealthy coping strategies or engage in actions that ultimately endanger their relationships' health.

Relationships that are not healthy frequently include;

Control, Disrespect, Dishonesty, Drama, Emotional abuse,Fear, Financial dishonesty or abuse Gaslighting, Guilt, Hostility, Intimidation, Isolation, Jealousy Loneliness, Negativity, Physical abuse, Poor communication, Ridicule Stress, Unhappiness Verbal abuse. Alternately, you might think that you always have to cover up what you really feel or think. You might even have the impression that in order to make the other person happy, you have to give up the things you really want.

The feeling that things are out of balance is another indication that the relationship is unhealthy. Relationships that are one-sided are those in which one person puts more effort, effort, and emotion into keeping the relationship going. Relationships of this kind can be unhealthy, and they frequently make the person who is doing all the work feel alone, unsupported, and depleted.

During times of extreme stress, unhealthy behaviors can occasionally emerge. In other instances, unhealthy behavior patterns that persist may worsen over time or emerge at various stages of a relationship.

Using self-help techniques or the assistance of a mental health professional, these issues can sometimes be resolved. But if there is physical, verbal, or sexual abuse in your relationship, your primary concern ought to be to ensure your safety.

Recap: Conflict or stress can sometimes bring about unhealthy patterns. Even though these are usually just temporary, more long-lasting unhealthy patterns mean that something needs to change or that the relationship may be ending. Because healthy relationships are so important to your well-being, it's important to protect yourself from those that could hurt your health. It is essential to resolve the issue if you believe you are in an unhealthy relationship. If both parties are committed to solving the issues and willing to change, change is possible.

What to do in an unhappy relationship.

1. <u>Determine Whether the unhealthy relationship Can Be Repaired.</u>

The first step is to determine whether the relationship can be repaired. It is necessary to ensure that both parties are willing to participate in making the relationship work in a way that is healthy for both parties involved in order to heal the damage and move forward. The relationship probably cannot be saved if one party refuses to alter their unhealthy behavior.

2. Maintain Interdependence Instead of encouraging codependency.

Healthy relationships encourage interdependence. Interdependent individuals comprehend the advantages of being able to turn to their partner when they require assistance and the significance and value of providing support for their partner. They are able to maintain their own sense of self outside of their relationship with their partner at the same time.

When two people in a relationship strive for interdependence, they are able to strike a balance that allows them to provide emotional intimacy and meet their partner's needs without becoming dependent on one another.

3. Establish a Strong Connection.

Establishing a strong connection with the other person is an essential step in ending a bad relationship. The following steps can help you overcome the unhealthy or toxic patterns that have been hurting your relationship and create a healthier, more supportive one. It is important to work together to overcome them.

Identify and avoid unhealthy patterns in your relationship by working together. Recognizing the problematic patterns that have been a problem for you both or any destructive behavior that has brought you to this point of disconnection is the first step toward developing a healthy emotional connection.

Make a list of the emotional needs that you value the most. It is essential to communicate these emotional goals for your relationship in order for there to be a genuine emotional understanding and emotional connection between you both. You cannot expect your partner to fulfill emotional needs that you do not make clear to them.

Offer your partner emotional support. Both of you need to be willing to provide positive emotional support that is free of guilt or manipulation in order for there to be an emotional connection between you and the other person.

When your partner speaks, pay close attention. Verbal communication is an essential component of emotional connection; therefore, ensure that you are supportive of these connections and cultivate them through meaningful conversation that demonstrates emotional interest, comprehension, and support.

Avoid manipulating your emotions. It is essential not to use the emotional connection as a means of coercing the other person into doing something they do not want to do. Doing so will only exacerbate the problems in your relationship and weaken the emotional connection you both share.

Other methods that may be of assistance:

Recap: There are steps you can take to address unhealthy patterns in a relationship.

1. Have personal goals and continue pursuing them.

2. Avoid minimizing yourself to please other people.

3. Focus on being your authentic self.

4. Spend time learning about what you like and what matters to you.

5. Expect others to treat you with respect.

6. Maintain your relationships with other people outside of the relationship.

7. If you decide that the relationship can be saved, find ways to maintain your dependence while building a strong emotional connection.

When to Get Help There are things you can do on your own to improve your relationship, but there are times when you may need the assistance of a mental health professional.

Couples therapy can help address issues in a relationship that are both personal and shared. A therapist, for instance, can assist in the treatment of underlying mental health issues that might be affecting how people relate to one another in a relationship.

When two people have different expectations of what they want from a relationship, a therapist can also help. In unhealthy one-sided relationships, for instance, one party may be responsible for more of the work because they are more invested, while the other party may be less invested.

Couples can also get help from a mental health professional working on improving their unhealthy communication skills, which can lead to toxicity and conflict in the relationship. A therapist can also assist each person in learning and practicing conflict management techniques.

Conflict can't be avoided, and it's not even a good idea. Even healthy relationships have disagreements and conflicts. Knowing how to handle it well is essential.

Recap: Therapy can be helpful if you are in an unhealthy relationship. When handled well, it allows people to address problems and make changes that are ultimately beneficial to the health of the relationship. A therapist can help you work on your own problems and learn new ways to deal with stress and communicate with others.When both parties are willing to participate and committed to making changes, therapy may be most beneficial.

When to Break Up with an Unhealthy Partner.

Not all relationships are worth keeping.If you've done your part but the other person isn't willing to change or help, it might be time to leave and work on building relationships that are healthier and more supportive.

Ending the relationship is frequently the most effective strategy for safeguarding your well-being if the other person has no desire to change or if the circumstance involves any form of abuse.

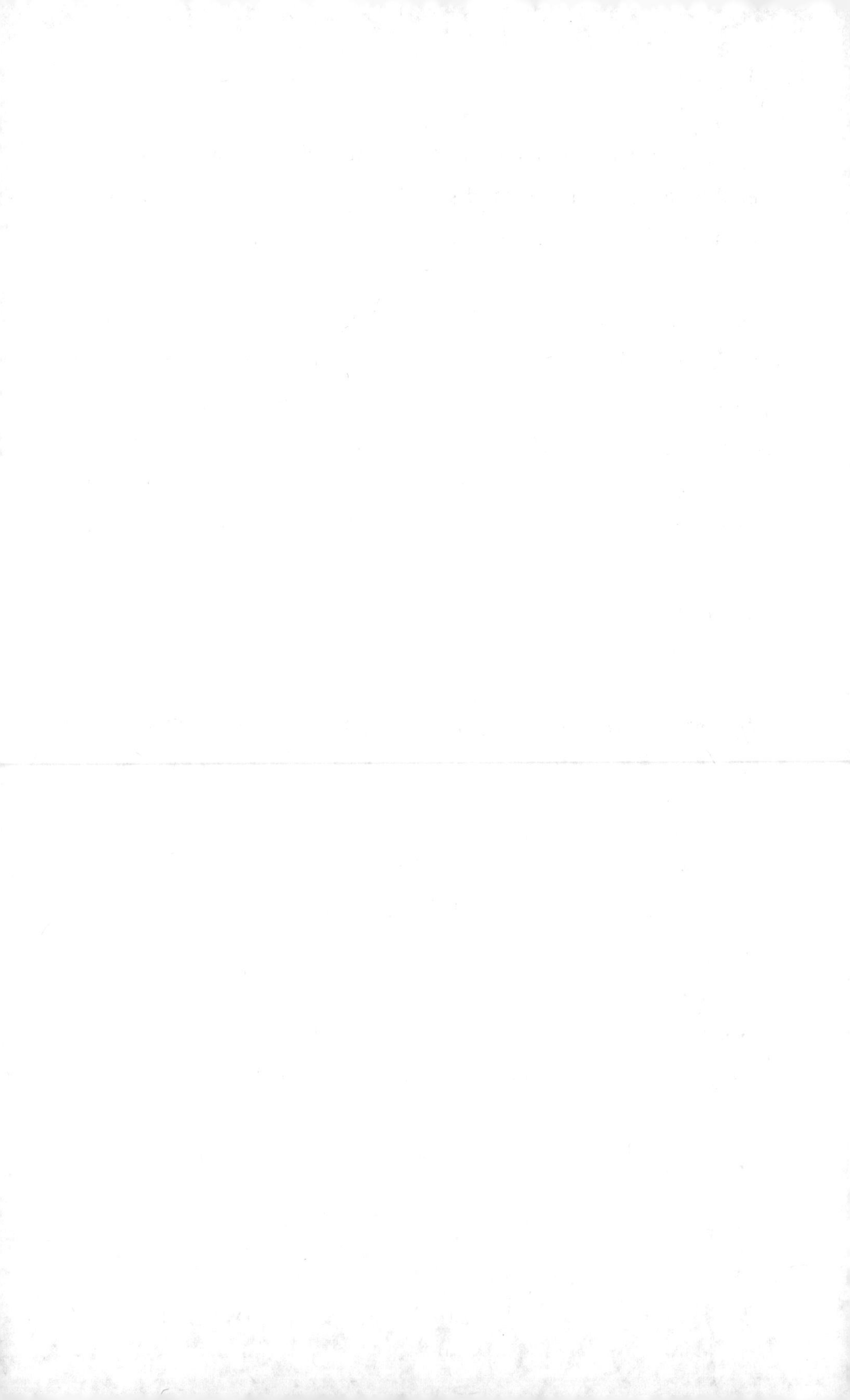